Title

Hope and healing

The fight against cancer

Kyle welch

How to Fight Cancer" is a powerful guide that offers inspiration and practical advice for those facing the difficult journey of cancer. From navigating the healthcare system to managing treatment side effects, this book provides a roadmap for finding hope and healing in the face of this devastating disease. With empathy, wisdom, and a deep understanding of the challenges facing cancer patients, "Hope and Healing: How to Fight Cancer" is an essential resource for anyone seeking to overcome this illness and emerge stronger on the other side."

Table contents

What is cancer?

Cancer is a term used to describe a group of diseases that involve abnormal cell growth. It is a leading cause of death worldwide and is caused by a variety of factors, including genetics, lifestyle, and environmental factors.

Cancer occurs when cells in the body divide and grow uncontrollably. This can lead to the formation of tumours, which can be either benign (non-cancerous) or malignant (cancerous).

Malignant tumours can spread to other parts of the body

The causes of cancer

The exact cause of cancer is not known, but there are several factors that can increase a person's risk of developing cancer. These include: smoking, excessive alcohol consumption, exposure to certain chemicals and radiation, a family history of cancer, a weakened immune system, and certain viruses and bacteria.

Symptoms of cancer:

Cancer is a disease that affects millions of people around the world every year. It is caused by abnormal cell growth that can spread to other parts of the body, leading to serious health complications and even death. While cancer can be a devastating diagnosis, it is important to understand that early detection and treatment can significantly improve your chances of survival.

One of the key factors in successfully treating cancer is catching it early. This is why regular cancer screenings are so important, especially if you have a family history of the disease or other risk factors. Depending on your age and gender, your doctor may recommend regular screenings for breast cancer, prostate cancer, colon cancer, cervical cancer, and other types of cancer.

In addition to regular screenings, it is important to be aware of the common signs and symptoms of cancer. These may include unexplained weight loss, persistent pain, changes in bowel or bladder habits, unusual bleeding, and persistent cough or hoarseness. If you experience any of these symptoms, it is important to talk to your doctor right away.

While there is no guaranteed way to prevent cancer, there are several steps you can take to reduce your risk. These may include maintaining a healthy weight, exercising regularly, eating a healthy diet, limiting alcohol consumption, avoiding tobacco products, and protecting your skin from the sun.

If you are diagnosed with cancer, it is important to remember that you are not alone. There are many resources available to help you through the treatment process, including support groups, counselling services, and cancer-specific organisations.

By understanding the importance of cancer awareness, regular screenings, and healthy lifestyle choices, you can take control of your health and reduce your risk of developing this devastating disease. Remember, early detection and treatment can save live

Cancer can present a wide range of symptoms, and the symptoms can vary depending on the type and stage of cancer. Some cancers may not cause any symptoms at all, while others can cause noticeable changes in your body that you should pay attention to.

Here are some common symptoms of cancer that you should be aware of:

Unexplained weight loss: Losing weight without trying can be a sign of several types of cancer, including pancreatic, stomach, lung, and colon cancer.

Persistent pain: Chronic pain that does not go away with medication or treatment can be a symptom of bone, brain, and other types of cancer.

Changes in bowel or bladder habits: Frequent diarrhoea, constipation, blood in the stool, or urinary incontinence can be signs of colon, bladder, or prostate cancer.

Unusual bleeding or discharge: Any unexplained bleeding or discharge, such as bleeding between periods or after menopause, can be a symptom of cervical, ovarian, or breast cancer.

Persistent cough or hoarseness: A cough that does not go away or becomes chronic can be a symptom of lung cancer, while hoarseness can be a symptom of throat or laryngeal cancer.

Skin changes: Changes in the colour, size, or shape of a mole, or the appearance of a new spot or lump on the skin, can be a symptom of skin cancer.

Fatigue: Feeling unusually tired or weak for no apparent reason can be a symptom of several types of cancer, including leukaemia and lymphoma.

It is important to note that many of these symptoms can also be caused by other health conditions that are not cancer-related. However, if you experience any of these symptoms, it is important to talk to your doctor as soon as possible to rule out the possibility of cancer or any other serious health condition. Early detection and treatment can make a significant difference in the outcome of cancer treatment, so it is important to pay attention to your body and seek medical attention if you notice any changes or symptoms. Fighting Cancer on Amazon.

Prevention: Encourage customers to make lifestyle changes that can help prevent cancer, such as eating a healthy diet, exercising regularly, not smoking, and avoiding excessive sun exposure.

Early detection: Encourage customers to get regular cancer screenings and checkups, such as mammograms, colonoscopies, and skin exams, to catch cancer early when it is most treatable.

Treatment options: Inform customers about different cancer treatment options available, including chemotherapy, radiation therapy, immunotherapy, surgery, and alternative therapies such as acupuncture or meditation.

Support resources: Inform customers about cancer support groups and resources, including online forums, counselling, and financial assistance programs.

Cancer research: Encourage customers to support cancer research through donations or participation in clinical trials, and to stay informed about the latest advances in cancer treatment and prevention.

Remember to always encourage your customers to consult with their healthcare provider before making any changes to their health routine.

How is cancer detected

There are several ways that cancer can be detected, including:

Screening tests: Screening tests are used to detect cancer before symptoms appear. Examples of screening tests include mammograms for breast cancer, Pap tests for cervical cancer, colonoscopies for colon cancer, and PSA tests for prostate cancer.

Imaging tests: Imaging tests, such as X-rays, CT scans, MRI scans, and PET scans, can be used to look for signs of cancer in the body.

Biopsy: A biopsy involves taking a sample of tissue from the suspicious area and examining it under a microscope to look for cancer cells.

Blood tests: Blood tests can be used to look for certain markers that may indicate the presence of cancer.

Physical exam: During a physical exam, a healthcare provider may check for lumps, changes in skin color, or other signs that may indicate the presence of cancer.

Living with cancer

1. Medical Care: Accessing the best medical care available, including specialists, treatments, and medications.

2. Emotional Support: Finding emotional support from family, friends, and support groups.

3. Financial Assistance: Seeking financial assistance to help cover medical costs and other expenses.

4. Nutrition and Exercise: Eating a healthy diet and engaging in regular physical activity.

5.ComplementaryTherapies:Exploring complementary therapies such as massage, yoga

The emotional toll of cancer

support resources

Cancer Support Groups: These are groups of people who have been affected by cancer, either directly or indirectly, and who meet regularly to provide emotional and practical support to one another.

Cancer Hotlines: These are telephone lines that provide information and emotional support to people affected by cancer.

Online Support Groups: These are online forums where people affected by cancer can connect with one another and share their experiences.

Ways of preventing Cancer

Cancer prevention tips.

I cannot make any guarantees about the effectiveness of any preventative measures. However, here are some general tips that may be helpful in reducing the risk of cancer for Amazon shoppers:

Maintain a healthy diet: Eating a healthy and balanced diet is one of the most important things you can do to reduce the risk of cancer. Try to eat plenty of fruits, vegetables, whole grains, lean proteins, and healthy fats, and limit processed and red meat, sugary drinks, and alcohol.

Exercise regularly: Regular physical activity can help reduce the risk of several types of cancer. Try to aim for at least 30 minutes of moderate exercise most days of the week.

Avoid tobacco: Smoking and other tobacco products increase the risk of several types of cancer, including lung, throat, and bladder cancer. If you smoke, quitting is one of the best things you can do for your health.

Protect your skin from the sun: Exposure to ultraviolet (UV) radiation from the sun can increase the risk of skin cancer. Use sunscreen with an SPF of at least 30, wear protective clothing, and avoid spending too much time in the sun during peak hours.

Get vaccinated: Certain viruses, such as human papillomavirus (HPV) and hepatitis B, can increase the risk of certain types of cancer. Vaccines are available for these viruses and can help prevent infection.

Get regular cancer screenings: Screening tests can help detect cancer early, when it is most treatable. Talk to your doctor about what types of screenings are recommended for your age and gender.

cancer awareness
"Cancer Awareness Matters"

Cancer is a disease that affects millions of people around the world every year. It is caused by abnormal cell growth that can spread to other parts of the body, leading to serious health complications and even death. While cancer can be a devastating diagnosis, it is important to understand that early detection and treatment can significantly improve your chances of survival.

One of the key factors in successfully treating cancer is catching it early. This is why regular cancer screenings are so important, especially if you have a family history of the disease or other risk factors. Depending on your age and gender, your doctor may recommend regular screenings for breast cancer, prostate cancer, colon cancer, cervical cancer, and other types of cancer.

In addition to regular screenings, it is important to be aware of the common signs and symptoms of cancer. These may include unexplained weight loss, persistent pain, changes in bowel or bladder habits, unusual bleeding, and persistent cough or hoarseness. If you experience any of these symptoms, it is important to talk to your doctor right away.

While there is no guaranteed way to prevent cancer, there are several steps you can take to reduce your risk. These may include maintaining a healthy weight, exercising regularly, eating a healthy diet, limiting alcohol consumption, avoiding tobacco products, and protecting your skin from the sun.

If you are diagnosed with cancer, it is important to remember that you are not alone. There are many resources available to help you through the treatment process, including support groups, counselling services, and cancer-specific organisations.

By understanding the importance of cancer awareness, regular screenings, and healthy lifestyle choices, you can take control of your health and reduce your risk of developing this devastating disease. Remember, early detection and treatment can save lives.

Cancer Caregiving

Cancer caregiving is the act of providing physical, emotional, and social support to someone who has been diagnosed with cancer. This type of care can be provided by family members, friends, or professional caregivers. Cancer caregiving can be a challenging and rewarding experience, as it involves providing support to someone who is going through a difficult time and helping them to manage their symptoms and treatment.

Some of the key responsibilities of a cancer caregiver include:

Providing emotional support: Cancer can be a very emotional experience, and caregivers can help by providing a listening ear, offering words of encouragement, and helping their loved one to stay positive.

Assisting with medical care: Caregivers may need to help with medication management, wound care, and other medical needs.

Managing household tasks: Caregivers may need to take on additional responsibilities around the house, such as cooking, cleaning, and running errands.

Advocating for their loved one: Caregivers may need to help their loved one navigate the healthcare system, communicate with doctors, and make important decisions about their care.

Providing transportation: Caregivers may need to help their loved one get to and from appointments and treatments.

Cancer caregiving can be a demanding and stressful role, and caregivers may experience burnout or other mental health issues as a result. It's important for caregivers to take care of themselves and seek support when needed. This can include talking to a therapist, joining a support group, or taking breaks from caregiving responsibilities.

Paediatric cancer

Paediatric cancer is a type of cancer that affects children and adolescents. It is the leading cause of death by disease in children under the age of 15 in the United States. Common types of Paediatric cancer include leukaemia, lymphoma, brain tumours, neuroblastoma, and Wilms tumour. Treatment for paediatric cancer typically involves a combination of surgery, chemotherapy, radiation therapy, and/or targeted therapy.

understanding and coping with childhood cancer

Childhood cancer is a devastating diagnosis for both the child and their family. Coping with the diagnosis, treatment, and aftermath of childhood cancer can be incredibly challenging. Here are some ways to understand and cope with childhood cancer:

Educate yourself: Learning about childhood cancer can help you understand what your child is going through and what to expect during treatment. Talk to your child's healthcare team, read books, and visit reputable websites to learn more about childhood cancer.

Find support: It is important to have a strong support system when dealing with childhood cancer. Reach out to family, friends, and support groups for help. Your child's healthcare team can also provide information about support groups and counselling services.

Take care of yourself: Caring for a child with cancer can be emotionally and physically exhausting. Make sure you take care of yourself by eating well, getting enough rest, and finding time to relax and recharge.

Communicate with your child: It is important to talk openly and honestly with your child about their diagnosis and treatment. Encourage your child to express their feelings and concerns, and listen to them with compassion.

Stay positive: While childhood cancer can be a difficult journey, it is important to stay positive and hopeful. Celebrate small victories and focus on the progress your child is making.

Keep a routine: Keeping a routine can help provide a sense of stability and normalcy for your child. Try to maintain regular meal times, bedtimes, and school schedules as much as possible.

Advocate for your child: Be an advocate for your child's needs and rights. Work closely with your child's healthcare team to ensure they receive the best possible care and treatment

.Cancer Risk Factors & Testing

The familiar risk factors and genetic testing of cancer

Cancer is a complex disease that can have both environmental and genetic factors. Some risk factors for cancer are well-known and established, while others are still being studied. Here are some familiar risk factors and genetic testing of cancer:

Age: The risk of developing cancer increases with age. Most cancer cases are diagnosed in people who are 55 years or older.

Family history: A family history of cancer can increase your risk of developing cancer. If your close relatives, such as parents or siblings, have had certain types of cancer, you may be at a higher risk for developing the same type of cancer.

Lifestyle factors: Certain lifestyle factors such as smoking, excessive alcohol consumption, poor diet, lack of physical activity, and exposure to environmental toxins can increase the risk of cancer.

Genetic mutations: Some genetic mutations can increase the risk of cancer. For example, mutations in the BRCA1 and BRCA2 genes increase the risk of breast and ovarian cancer.

Genetic testing: Genetic testing can identify certain genetic mutations that increase the risk of cancer. Testing is typically done in individuals who have a family history of a certain type of cancer, or who have been diagnosed with cancer at a young age.

Do not panic

Cancer is a serious disease, but it is not always a death sentence. With advances in cancer research and treatment, many types of cancer are curable or can be managed as a chronic condition.

Early detection and treatment are key to improving cancer outcomes. Regular cancer screenings, such as mammograms or colonoscopies, can help detect cancer at an early stage when it is most treatable.

There are many different treatments available for cancer, including surgery, chemotherapy, radiation therapy, targeted therapy, and immunotherapy. The choice of treatment depends on the type and stage of cancer, as well as the individual's overall health and preferences.

While there are no guarantees with cancer treatment, many people with cancer are able to live long, fulfilling lives after treatment. It's important to have a positive attitude and to seek support from loved ones and healthcare professionals during this challenging time.

In conclusion, cancer is not always a death sentence and it is possible to recover from or manage the disease. Regular screenings, early detection, and advances in cancer treatment have led to improved outcomes for many people with cancer.

A PET CT scan is a medical imaging technique that combines two different types of scans, namely a Positron Emission Tomography (PET) scan and a Computed Tomography (CT) scan. PET scans use a small amount of radioactive material called a radiotracer to detect changes in cellular metabolism and activity, while CT scans use X-rays to create detailed images of the internal structures of the body.

During a PET CT scan, the patient is injected with a radiotracer, which is a radioactive compound that is designed to accumulate in specific tissues or organs of the body. The radiotracer emits positrons, which are detected by a PET scanner to create a three-dimensional image of the metabolic activity of the tissue.

The CT scan is then performed to provide additional information on the location and size of any abnormalities detected by the PET scan. The CT images are combined with the PET images to create a highly detailed, three-dimensional image that provides information about the function and structure of the tissue being imaged.

PET CT scans are commonly used in the diagnosis and management of cancer, as they can detect cancerous cells and tumors in the body. They can also be used to monitor the effectiveness of cancer treatments, such as chemotherapy or radiation therapy, and to detect the recurrence of cancer after treatment.

Overall, PET CT scans are a valuable diagnostic tool that can provide detailed information about the structure and function of tissues and organs in the body, which can be used to guide treatment decisions and improve patient outcomes.